Proven

OBESITY

CODE

A detailed guide to unlocking the
secrets of losing weight and
never gaining it back

Dr. Jason Fred

Disclaimer

This book is designed to provide information about the subject matter covered. It was sold with an understanding that the publisher and author were not rendering professional services of any kind. If expert assistance is required, then it should be sought first and foremost from a competent professional who can offer you appropriate guidance on your particular needs before considering anything else contained within the pages of this guide. Every effort has been made to make this book as complete and accurate as possible. However, there may still exist mistakes both in typography (spelling) errors and also content-wise which will hopefully be corrected by future editions if necessary.

The stories outlined within this book, while based in part on fact, have been modified so as not to reveal the identity of any real person. Any resemblance between people depicted in this book either living or dead persons is strictly coincidental. The purpose of this book is to enlighten, inspire, and entertain the reader.

Neither author nor publisher shall be liable for damages caused directly or indirectly by information presented herein.

Table of Contents

INTRODUCTION

The idea of losing weight and keeping it off is a dream for many people. However, it quickly becomes a nightmare when the weight returns.

This is because some people who lose weight don't understand what causes them to gain it back and subsequently fall into cycles of yo-yo dieting. They often turn to quick fixes that only provide temporary results, which leads them right back where they started from: overweight with no idea how to get out of their self-created mess.

Losing weight and keeping it off seems like such a difficult task, but the truth is that you can do it!

It is not your fault if you haven't found success in losing weight before; there are just so many things going on behind the scenes that we're unaware of! It can be tough for anyone looking for a way to finally shed pounds once and for all - but now that you have hidden secrets at your disposal, I hope you have more success in your weight-loss journey than ever before.

CHAPTER ONE

WHAT YOU HAVE BEEN MISSING IN YOUR WEIGHT LOSS JOURNEY

There is an old saying that goes: "If you don't know where you're going, you won't get anywhere"

I talk to a lot of people who want to reduce their weight and one of the first things I ask them is, "How much weight do you want to lose?" The usual response I get looks like:

"Oh, I don't know, I just want to get rid of my excess weight" or "I'm just trying to lose some weight" ...

In fact, I believe that the majority of people I talk to don't know exactly how badly they want to reduce their weight! Or they just have an idea of how much to lose, but it's a number given to them by maybe some doctor, personal trainer, or some chart, and not what they personally want to lose.

When you pair this lack of clarity on the weight loss goal with the fact that 95% of people who want to reduce their weight are never successful in the long term, you start to see the big picture.

Surprisingly too, a number of these people also don't know exactly how much they weigh in the first place - since they avoid stepping on a scale. How do you know if you're successful if you don't even know where you're starting out or where you want to go?

The simple answer is, you cannot succeed!

If you were on a trip and needed to get to a specific place you had never been before, do you want to leave like that blindly and hope to get there? No! Of course, you wouldn't.

In order to plot an effective route, you need to indicate your starting point and destination, in order to determine the distance, the best route, whether you need to travel by car, plane or boat, what time you need to leave, how long will it take you, and so on ...

You can use Google Maps, or you can phone where you're going, so they can give you directions, or ask someone who's been there before. Either way, you need to have a clear destination in mind.

Do you see where I am going with this?

If you can plan a trip in so much detail to get to where you want to go, what is stopping you from planning your "weight reduction trip" in a similar way and giving yourself the best chance of getting there? Achieving the weight you want to be?

The answer could be that you don't really know where to start.

The first thing you need to do is to find out where you are now! It means weighing yourself and understanding your current state of health. Many people who are overweight generally dislike weighing themselves, but it is an essential part of your weight loss journey. So, do it.

Proven Obesity Code

After you have found out where you are, you then have to decide on your end result! Determine for yourself the reasonable weight you would like to achieve. Make sure it is achievable and that it is a healthy weight for you. You now know by how much you need to reduce your weight.

Losing weight is the type of decision that you can't just put your foot in the water with. You need to dive head, body and soul.

When you commit to your weight loss decision, there is enthusiasm, motivation and courage to keep your efforts going until the end. If you are not really committed, it will be more difficult to reach your goal because the fact is that it is not an easy process. Eating your favorite cake is certainly more pleasurable.

There is no doubt about the importance of being truly committed to weight loss, but it is also true that many people simply cannot commit.

Start and don't stop! Sorry if that sounds simple, but we hear so many people saying "I'm going to start next week" or "I'm just taking a day off, I'll be back tomorrow." It's a harsh reality and you can't afford to stop every now and then or take a "week (or month!) Off". There is no better time to start than now, and no better time to quit until you are fully successful.

Proven Obesity Code

CHAPTER TWO

HOW TO NEVER GIVE UP IN YOUR WEIGHT LOSS JOURNEY

One of the biggest challenges people face when it comes to losing weight is Motivation. Indeed, even if you know how to lose weight, knowing how to find the motivation to change your habits can be another story!

A weight loss journey seldom follows a linear trajectory: you may have to deal with losses, gains, and plateaus. In order to stay motivated through the ups and downs, set goals that are unrelated to weight.

This will give you other ways to measure your progress. Growth is a basic human need. We need to feel that we are improving our life.

If you have set your target weight, planned your exercise program and finally decided to join the sports club near you. Now you just need to maintain that level of enthusiasm throughout your diet. While losing weight can seem like a daunting and difficult task, a few simple techniques can help you stay motivated for the long haul.

If you're wondering how to stay motivated to lose weight, start by figuring out your why.

Many people start to lose weight because they have to. Losing weight under your doctor's recommendation can be a good start, but the best motivation comes from within. Dig deep and determine why you actually want to lose weight.

Some of your reasons may be:

- Have more self-confidence,
- A need for recognition,
- To please your partner,

Whatever the reasons, personal or professional, I invite you to go deeper into your thinking and think about what weight loss could change in your life.

Also, it is possible to consult with your healthcare provider for weight, height, and weight-related risk factors. Make a follow-up appointment to monitor changes in your weight or health-related situations.

Keep a "food diary" for a few days, where you write down everything you eat. This journal allows you to be more aware of what you eat and when you eat it. By being aware of this you can avoid mindlessly eating.

Then take a look at your current lifestyle. Identify obstacles that can hinder your weight loss efforts.

For example, does your work schedule or travel prevent you from getting enough physical activity?

Do you tend to eat sugar-rich foods because that's what you buy for your children?

Do your coworkers often bring high-calorie foods to share, like donuts?

Think about what you can do to overcome these challenges.

Think about the aspects of your lifestyle that can help you lose weight.

For example, is there an area near your work where you and your colleagues can go for a walk after lunch?

Is there a place in your community, like the YMCA, with sports facilities for you and childcare services for your children?

Once you know the "why" of your project, I now invite you to set a realistic goal. Saying "I want to lose 20 pounds in two weeks" is just unrealistic and might put you off. For example, you can already begin to determine your ideal weight which you can use to benchmark and adjust it according to your will.

Set some short-term goals and reward your efforts throughout the process. If your long-term goal is to lose 40 pounds and control your high blood pressure, you can set short-term eating and physical activity goals such as starting breakfast, taking a 15-minute walk at night, or eating salad or vegetables for dinner.

Focus on two or three goals at a time. The most effective goals are:

- Concrete
- Realistic
- Comprehensive (we are not perfect)

For example, "exercising more" is not a specific goal. But if you say "I am going to walk 15 minutes, 3 days a week in the first week," you are setting a concrete and realistic goal for the first week.

Remember, small changes every day leads to big results in the long run. Also remember that realistic goals are achievable goals. By reaching short-term goals day by day, you feel good about your progress and motivated to continue. Setting unrealistic goals, such as losing 20 pounds in 2 weeks, brings feelings of defeat and frustration.

Being realistic also means knowing that there may be setbacks. Setbacks happen when you go off plan for whatever reason, such as holidays, working longer hours, or going through another change in your life.

When you experience a setback, try to resume your plan as soon as possible. Also take some time to think about what you would do differently if faced with a similar situation, to avoid setbacks.

Keep in mind that everyone is different: what works for some, does not work for others. Even if your neighbor has lost weight just by running, it doesn't mean that running is the best option for you. Try a variety of physical activities that you enjoy the most and that are compatible with your life, such as walking, swimming, playing tennis, or taking group exercise classes. It will be easier for you to continue doing these activities in the long term.

Always make sure to keep an eye on its progress. Different methods can be used to follow its evolution (weight, fat mass rate, measurements, photos).

If you have a stroke of the blues, I invite you for example to consult the evolution of your weight. Seeing that you have already lost 5.10 or even 15 kilos prove to you that you are of course on the right path and that with persistence and determination, you will succeed in achieving your goals.

It is also important that you review the goals you set for yourself and assess your progress on a regular basis. If you make a goal to walk every morning but have a hard time doing it before you go to work, consider changing your work schedule or try going for a walk at lunchtime or after work.

Evaluate which parts of your plan are working well and which parts need adjustment. Then rewrite your goals and plan based on this assessment.

If you are consistently achieving your goals, keep adding goals to stay on the road to success.

That being said, it is time to find yourself a partner who will support you in your fight against extra pounds. As we often say, there is strength in unity. It's easier to give up and find excuses not to move your butt when you're alone.

Together, it will be possible to motivate and encourage each other. You will create a real team spirit and have a better chance of staying on track.

We often say that we are the average of the 5 people we hang out with the most. Surround yourself with successful people, who play sports, who take care of their health. These people will have a positive impact on you.

If you really don't have people around you to support you in your project, it is always possible to search the internet for a group that has the same objective as you. For this, there are social networks such as Facebook or forums specializing in weight loss. Having virtual friends is always better than nothing.

Celebrate your successes as you progress

Losing weight is difficult, so celebrate all of your successes to stay motivated.

Give yourself credit when you accomplish a goal. Social media or some community pages specializing in weight loss are great places to share your successes and get help. Do not hesitate to talk about it around you and be proud of your results.

Celebrate changes and achieved goals. For example, if your goal this week was to lose 1 pound, reward yourself with a good bubble bath, for example, or plan a fun night out with friends.

Then take it to the next level by setting other goals. For example, increase the intensity or duration of your sports sessions.

However, it is important to choose your rewards wisely. Avoid rewarding yourself with food. Also, avoid expensive rewards and focus on simple activities instead.

Here are some good examples of rewards:

-       A manicure

- Go to the movies
- Buy a new top for your workouts
- Take a cooking class

Don't be too hard on yourself

Make a weight loss plan that's right for you and that you can stick to for the long haul. It is the diet that should adapt to you and not the other way around. Although there are hundreds of different diets, most are based on calorie reduction.

While reducing your calorie intake will lead to weight loss, it is not necessarily recommended to follow a diet, as diets often tend to ban certain foods altogether. Therefore, those with a "weaker" state of mind will tend to crack more easily and be less likely to lose weight.

Instead, consider creating your own personalized plan and adopting healthy eating habits that are free to boycott certain foods. This will be much more effective in the long term and will avoid the "yo-yo" effect.

Sometimes it is good to be firm in your goals and work hard to achieve them. But it's also important to be forgiving. Losing weight is no easy task and no need to develop additional stress.

Also, learn to love your body. Make sure you appreciate your body throughout your weight loss journey. Focusing on activities that make us feel competent and strong and thinking about what we particularly value about our body can help.

For example, even if you are not thrilled by the sight of your arms in the mirror, you can focus on the fact that these arms allow you to hug your children tightly against you. To prevent a drop in motivation, get used to taking note of what your body is capable of on a regular basis - perhaps every morning while brushing your teeth or while stretching at the end of your workout. It is yet another motivating reminder that this course is much more than a story of weight.

Life is a journey, don't expect everything to be easy. Weight loss is part of that journey. If you've stepped off the bandwagon, don't wait until the next New Year to set foot there again. Today can be the new day.

Staying motivated to lose weight isn't always easy. Despite everything, it is possible to work on your motivation. It is about adopting certain tricks and knowing how to change your mentality. Your motivation can be compared to fueling a car. When it is empty, it will be difficult to move forward!

CHAPTER THREE

WAYS TO REACH YOUR WEIGHT LOSS GOALS EASILY

Many people start some kind of activity, practice for some time and then stop; and they usually do this more than once. Generally, the main reason is anxiety and frustration at not getting the expected results.

It is necessary to be aware that the results do not appear overnight. In order to achieve goals, you must be focused, predisposed to change, leave behind old habits and have enough discipline to incorporate new ones. After all, for an activity to effectively become a habit in our routine, it is necessary that we perform it several times.

That notwithstanding, here are some of the ways to easily attain your weight loss goals:

Increasing Your Daily Steps Will Help You Lose Weight

Walking 10,000 steps per day, which equals about five miles or 8.5 kilometers on average (depending on the size of the steps) contributes to overall health and can help with weight control.

The 10,000 step goal is a goal set by the American Heart Association to promote cardiovascular health. This is not an "absolute" or "pass/fail" course of action, but a number that sets a useful benchmark.

If you want to start training or come back from an injury, you'll want to start slowly to avoid further injury or becoming overly fatigued. It is helpful to wear a fitness tracker or pedometer to determine how many steps you take on average each day over the course of a week. This becomes your starting point. It's generally recommended that you add 1,000 daily steps at a time, so if your baseline is 3,000 steps per day, set your new goal to 4,000 steps per day.

Unless you have a very active lifestyle or profession, you probably won't achieve the 10,000 steps per day without putting extra effort into planning walks or other activities. For most people, achieving 10,000 steps a day is a good goal, because it's convenient, free, and simple to achieve with just a small tweak to your daily routine.

However, since it can seem difficult to walk 10,000 steps, it is important that you develop a strategy to meet your daily quota. Here are three easy ways to help you achieve your goals without losing focus:

Use a pedometer or fitness tracker

Using a pedometer can help you easily track how far you've walked throughout your day as well as the number of steps you've taken. A pedometer is a small, box-shaped calculator that you can hang from your belt or pants pocket in the same way you wear a pager. When placed firmly near the hip, the pedometer records every step you take.

For people who want to meet their new daily step quota, the pedometer or fitness tracker are easy and reliable tools to assess your progress towards your goal. When shopping for a pedometer, be sure to select a model that shows both distance and number of steps.

Fitness trackers are typically worn around the wrist. They are relatively inexpensive and fairly accurate. Some come with additional features like measuring your heart rate which allows you to track the number of calories you burn, as well as the level of intensity of the exercise you do which are "advanced" features that go beyond to count steps.

By tracking your daily steps, you will begin to learn how many steps go in a kilometer or a mile. You'll also be amazed at how many steps you can add to your daily count by changing little habits, like choosing the stairs instead of the elevator or walking to your colleague's desk rather than emailing.

Calculate the time it takes

For example, if you know that you can reach your step goal in an hour, then you can choose to dedicate an hour every day to get your steps. However, if you can't devote a full hour, you can add ten minutes increments at a time until you reach your goal. Having a clear understanding of what it takes to reach your goal will help you approach the task much more strategically than if you didn't have a plan. Do the math to save time and make sure you hit your daily goal.

Measure a route

Measure a route based on the time and distance it takes to reach your goal. Having a pre-planned route will help you see the task and reach your target in a more manageable way. You will be able to measure your progress during the day and have a system to achieve your goals. Because taking the same route every day can get tedious, plan two or three alternative routes.

Plan a long route for the days when you have tons of energy, a short route for the days when you are tired, and a mid-route route for the days when you are energetic, but busy. Giving yourself plenty of options is important in helping you stay positive and enthusiastic so that you can achieve your long-term goals.

10,000 steps a day might not make sense to you at first. You may need to plan fewer steps per day if you are not in good shape, and conversely, you may need to walk more if you want to lose a lot of weight.

Your step goal may vary based on your needs, and it may also change over time. For starters, 10,000 steps a day is a good target for most of us struggling to lose weight and get healthy.

Go ahead and try it for a month and see what it will do for you. One thing is for sure, you will be healthier and happier.

Team up with like minds at school or work to lose weight faster

Have you heard the old saying "the fastest way to get to where you want to go is to help someone else get there"?

According to a study published in the Journal of Consulting and Clinical Psychology, teaming up at school or work to lose weight may be one of the best ways to achieve your diet goals. The study followed a group of friends who joined together in an effort to lose weight as well as several individuals with similar goals. At the end of the study, the researchers found that people who teamed up were not only more likely to complete their diet program, but also to lose more weight than people who dieted without a supportive partner. Additionally, partners who dieted were more successful in maintaining weight loss than those who dieted on their own.

So, what makes the big difference between dieting with a partner and dieting alone? Researchers believe that the element of social support is a compelling factor. A weight loss partner can provide both the moral support and the discipline you need to stay on track.

While just about anyone can be a weight loss partner, researchers believe that school or work buddies are better weight loss partners because they are not as likely to pass on judgments like family member or even close friends. Additionally, a school or work weight loss partner is more likely to understand the unique frustrations dieters face in the real world of work or school.

When making the decision to team up at work or school, you should consider several key factors when choosing a weight loss partner. One of the first factors you should consider is the type of weight loss partner that would best meet your needs. For example, ask yourself if you need someone to exercise with you anymore or someone to help you avoid dessert-laden office nights and the ritual afternoon snack?

You should also consider finding a partner who will blend in well with your personality as well as your schedule and workplace. Even if you work for the same company as someone else interested in losing weight; if your schedules are constantly in conflict, there's a good chance you won't be able to support each other. The same goes when looking for a weight loss partner in school; the buddy system will work much better if your schedules are similar and if the classes are located close to each other.

Finally, be sure to seek out a weight loss partner who is not too strict or too forgiving in their support. Look for someone who will support you, but who will be firm in keeping you on track.

When you find the right supportive partner, be sure to sit down with them to discuss common goals. Think about ways you can support each other in your weight loss efforts, like these:

- Take turns bringing healthy snacks to work or school.

- Set aside a time of the day when you can discuss progress, failures and tips.
- Gather to visit the gym, take an aerobics class or take a walk during lunchtime.
- Swap recipes that are low in calories, fat or carbs.
- Mutually celebrate victories.

You can do this if you plan and eat the right foods and stay active while having the right support. And whatever you do, don't procrastinate. Procrastination only turns a good plan into a failure. When you wait to do something, it usually doesn't happen. There is only one thing left for you to do: cheer on your partner and start!

Avoid eating for the wrong reasons due to social influence

Many obese or overweight people get this condition because they don't have the right relationship with food. They can use the food for comfort when they are sad or to occupy themselves when they are not busy. Still others eat for pleasure. Look at the way we entertain our friends. It's all about food.

We usually meet our friends for dinner at a restaurant or invite them to a feast at home. It's all about food and a lot of food. This is a real problem because when you think of food this way, it's hard to change what you eat.

If you don't eat to provide the right kind of food for your body, you will be trapped in this pitfall. Food is primarily supposed to be fuel for your body to function. But if food becomes your main source of entertainment and pleasure, things can go off the rails.

It takes time, work, and sometimes the help of a professional psychologist, but you need to make sure that you are eating for the right reasons. Food should be viewed as a tool you use to lose weight, not as social entertainment or emotional support.

Think about the people you spend the most time with, and it is likely that some of them weigh about the same, if not more, than you. When everyone around you invites you to eat unhealthy foods and encourages you to forget about your diet just for tonight, it's easy to give in and keep giving in until you've lost track of your diet completely.

Sometimes you may need to cut ties with certain people around you or at least spend less time with them so that you can focus on what you need to do and not let their negative influences affect you. You can also try to take the initiative when it comes to planning activities and suggest that your meetings include more physical activity or healthy restaurants.

The next time you plan to get together with friends, try meeting them for a nice walk in the park or a bike ride on the bike path. Chances are you'd have more fun than just sitting around a table and getting drunk from plate to plate.

If you want to lose weight, you will need to make choices and make lifestyle changes. You can even influence your friends for the better.

CHAPTER FOUR

LIFESTYLES AND HABITS FOR A SMOOTHER WEIGHT LOSS JOURNEY

If you recently lost excess weight, congratulations! This achievement will likely benefit your present and future health. Now that you've lost weight, let's talk about some ways to avoid getting it back.

The tips below reflect common characteristics of people who have been able to lose weight without regaining it over time.

1.Watch your diet

A healthy lifestyle has started, now the challenge is to maintain the positive eating habits adopted along the way. In studies of people who lost weight and did not regain it for at least a year, most of them continued to eat a lower calorie diet compared to what they ate before dieting.

Keep your eating patterns consistent and eat breakfast every day. Follow a healthy eating pattern regardless of changes in your routine. Plan ahead for weekends, vacations, and special occasions. By having a plan, you are more likely to have healthy foods on hand for when you change your routine.

Eating breakfast is a common practice for people who have lost weight and have not regained it. A healthy breakfast can help you avoid building up hunger and overeating later.

When it comes to eating, we all have very ingrained habits. Some are good ("I always have my breakfast") and others are not so good ("I always leave my plate clean"). Although many eating habits are acquired from childhood, it does not mean that it is too late to change them.

Sudden and radical changes in eating habits, such as eating nothing but cabbage soup, can lead to short-term weight loss. But these exaggerated changes are neither healthy nor good and will not help in the long run. To permanently improve eating habits, a **Reflect, Substitute** and **Strengthen** approach is needed.

- **REFLECT** on all of your eating habits, both good and bad, as well as the things that trigger unhealthy eating.
- **SUBSTITUTE** your unhealthy eating habits with healthier ones.
- **STRENGTHEN** your new eating habits.

Reflect, Substitute, and Strengthen: A Process to Improve Your Eating Habits

Make a list of your eating habits. Keeping a "food diary" for a few days where you write down everything you eat and the time you eat will help you figure out your habits. For example, it may be that you always want something sweet when you feel your energy low in the middle of the afternoon. Use food diary to compile the list. It's good to write down how you felt when you decided to eat, especially if you weren't hungry. Were you tired or stressed?

Underline the habits on the list that are causing you to eat more than you need. Eating habits that can often lead to weight gain include:

- Eating very fast
- Eating everything that is served from the plate
- Eating when you are not hungry
- Eating standing up (can make you eat without thinking about what you eat or very quickly)
- Always eating dessert
- Skipping meals (or just breakfast)

Review the unhealthy eating habits you have highlighted. Be sure to identify all the factors that trigger those habits. Identify some of the ones you will try to change first. Be sure to congratulate yourself on the things you do well. Maybe you almost always eat fruit for dessert or drink low-fat or fat-free milk. These are good habits! By acknowledging your accomplishments, you will be motivated to make more changes.

Make a list of "triggers" by reviewing your food diary. You will be more aware of where and when "triggers" arise to eat without feeling hungry. Write down how you usually feel on those occasions. Often an environmental "trigger" or a particular mood is what prompts us to eat without feeling hungry. Common triggers that drive you to eat when you're not hungry:

- Open a drawer and find your favorite snack.
- Sit at home and watch television.
- Before or after a meeting or stressful situation at work.
- Coming home from work and having no idea what to eat.
- Have someone offer you a dish they made "just for you"!
- Pass a sweet dish on a counter.

- Sit in the lunchroom at work near the vending machine for treats or snacks.
- See a plate of donuts in the morning during a business meeting.
- Spend every morning at the window of your favorite fast food restaurant.
- Feeling bored or tired and thinking that eating something will lift your spirits.

Circle the "triggers" from the list that you face on a daily or weekly basis. Getting together with your family on Thanksgiving can be a "trigger" for overeating. It would be nice if you have a plan in place to counteract these factors. But for now, focus on the ones you have most often.

Ask yourself the following for each "trigger" factor you have circled:

- Is there anything I can do to avoid this trigger or situation? This option works best with some triggers that are independent of others. For example, could you take a different route to work to avoid stopping at your favorite fast food restaurant? Is there another place in the lunchroom at work where you can sit that is not near the vending machine?

- Of the things that I cannot avoid, can I do something different that is healthier? Obviously, you can't avoid all situations that trigger unhealthy eating habits, like work meetings. In these circumstances, evaluate your options. Could you suggest or bring healthy snacks and drinks? Could you offer to take notes to distract your attention from those snacks? Could you sit further away from the food so that it is not easy for you to grab something? Could you have a healthy snack before the meeting?

Replace unhealthy habits with new healthy habits. For example, as you reflect on your eating habits, you may find that you eat too quickly when you are alone. To counteract this, arrange to have lunch each week with a co-worker or invite a neighbor over for dinner one night a week. Other strategies may be to place the silverware on the plate between bites or to minimize other distractions (such as watching the news at dinner time) with which we cannot pay attention to the time it takes to eat or the amount of food.

Reinforce your new healthy habits and be patient with yourself. Habits are formed over time; they are not adopted overnight. When you see that you are practicing an unhealthy habit, quickly stop and ask yourself: Why am I doing this? When did I start to do it? What do I need to change? Don't be too hard on yourself or think that one mistake will ruin a whole day of healthy habits. You can do it! You can do it one day at a time!

Proven Obesity Code

Your body does not gain weight when the number of calories in the food you eat (the deposits) equals the amount of energy your body needs and uses to function (the withdrawals).

If you eat more calories than your body uses, the extra calories are stored as body fat. If you consume an additional 900 calories per day, when your body has already absorbed the calories it needs for that day, those 900 calories will be converted into 100 grams of fat, or almost a quarter of a pound (which accumulates in your bank account).

Eating healthy can help you lose and keep weight off. It is best to lose weight by making these healthy changes which can become new habits. It is common knowledge that excessively calorie restrictive diets are also more likely to fail. Even if they help you lose weight in the short term, you are more likely to get it back because you haven't changed your lifestyle.

2.Stay physically active

Get physical activity every day. People who have lost weight and have not regained it generally spend 60 to 90 minutes in moderate intensity physical activity almost every day of the week and do not consume more calories than they need. This does not necessarily mean 60 to 90 minutes in a single session. It can be 20 to 30 minutes of physical activity three times a day. For example, brisk walking in the morning, at lunchtime, and at night. Some people may need to consult with their doctor before engaging in this level of physical activity.

By "physical activity" I mean here any movement leading to energy expenditure. It can therefore be climbing stairs, walking your dog, or doing the dishes, or any practice making it possible to improve the physical condition, such as for example the musculation exercises allowing to develop the force, the long-distance races improving the endurance, or the stretching improving the flexibility.

Of course, by definition, physical exercises are part of the large family of physical activities, just like sports (for which the notion of competition is provided).

As you lose weight, more physical activity increases the number of calories your body "burns" or uses for energy. By burning calories through physical activity while reducing the number of calories you eat, you create a "caloric deficit" that results in weight loss.

Most of the weight is lost by eating fewer calories. However, evidence shows that the fastest way to maintain weight loss is to engage in regular physical activity.

Most importantly, physical activity reduces the risk of cardiovascular disease and diabetes to a greater extent than weight loss alone.

Physical activity also helps:

- Keep in weight.
- Reduce high blood pressure.

- Reduce the risk of type 2 diabetes, heart attack, stroke, and various types of cancer.
- Reduce arthritis pain and disability associated with this condition.
- Reduce the risk of osteoporosis and falls.
- Reduce symptoms of depression and anxiety.

3.Keep your course

Watch your diet and your activity. Keeping a journal of your food and your physical activity can help you track your progress and identify your trends. For example, you may notice that your weight increases during periods when you travel a lot for work or when you have to work overtime. Recognizing this tendency may indicate that you should try other behaviors, such as taking your own healthy meals for the plane or finding a little time to exercise in the gym of the hotel where you are staying on your trip. If you work overtime, you can take short walks around the building during breaks.

Watch your weight. Check your weight regularly. To control lost weight, it is a good idea to keep track of your weight in order to plan and adjust your exercise and eating plan as needed. If you gained a few pounds, correct this trend quickly.

Seek support from family, friends, and others. People who have successfully lost weight and have not regained it often rely on the support of others to stay on track and overcome setbacks. Sometimes having a friend or partner who is also losing weight or trying to maintain their new weight can help you stay motivated.

Are you not disillusioned with playing yo-yo with your weight? If you want to lose weight, you will have to make some new choices. Easier said than done! Sometimes we have to fight our own demons. If you find it too difficult, don't give up and throw in the towel... ask for help instead!

Dr. Jason Fred

CHAPTER FIVE

HOW TO PREVENT RELAPSES AND AVOID GAINING YOUR WEIGHT BACK

Most time, after losing weight, you remain "fragile" and engrossed in fear of being at risk of regaining the weight. Here, I'll explore the reasons for this fragility, and ways to help you prevent relapse.

A central issue in weight control, as it is with every other type of behavioral problem, is how to reduce the risk of relapse. In fact, it's not an exaggeration to say that reducing the risk of relapse is the primary task of treatment.

Many methods can initiate change, such as a week at a health spa (fun!) or a 21-day diet and exercise plan (not fun!), but these short-term interventions do not fix the long-term problem. Of course, the initial focus of all treatment is symptom reduction (losing the weight, stopping drinking, recovering from depression, etc.); this is the necessary first step.

You must lose the weight before you can confront the challenge of maintenance. However, you need to start preparing for maintenance before you get there and not take it for granted.

Thus, we often see people launch themselves into an intensive program, the more stringent the better, and get dramatic results. They feel happy, proud, and confident, but unfortunately, they go off course at some point, feel defeated and discouraged, lose focus, and find it difficult to get back on track.

No matter how well it seems to go during the initial intensive, "boot camp" phase, these individuals remain "fragile" with respect to their risk of relapse.

The reason for this fragility is two-fold:

First, the intensive regime is not physically or psychologically sustainable and does not represent a real lifestyle change. Real lifestyle changes are built from less dramatic small shifts in daily life that add up to big changes over time. Real lifestyle change requires you to deal with all the stresses and strains and competing demands of "your" life.

Second, diets do not teach people how to master the relapse crisis itself. This is another key challenge in long-term behavior change, and where psychology plays a very important role. It's learning to deal with, and indeed to learn from, the relapse crisis that is the key to lasting change and successful weight loss maintenance.

The most well-established model of relapse and relapse prevention was proposed about 40 years ago by a psychologist named Alan Marlatt. His initial work was with alcoholics, but the model has since been applied to all sorts of behavior change.

In the relapse prevention model, the first question is how one copes with a "high risk" situation. High risk situations are those that increase the likelihood of an initial "lapse" (a slip back to the old behavior) for an individual; these high-risk situations often involve negative emotions and interpersonal situations, but may also involve positive events such as parties, holidays, and celebrations.

When we face such a situation, we are challenged to find a way to cope. If we manage to cope successfully, we gain knowledge and confidence, and reduce our future risk of relapse. On the other hand, if we fail to cope, giving in to temptation and deviating from our plans, we may lose confidence and become even more prone to relapse.

Importantly, even a failure to cope can lead to learning, as we come up with strategies to avoid or cope with similar situations in the future. Thus, it is not just the occurrence of a lapse that is important, but how it is interpreted. If a lapse is interpreted negatively ("I knew this would happen, changing my bad habits is impossible!"), it can lead to a spiral of bad behavior and loss of motivation ("what the hell, I've blown it, so I may as well continue....at least I'll have the pleasure of eating").

If one's confidence is shaken beyond a certain point of no return, we are likely to conclude that further efforts are pointless and quit. It is as if each time we face a high-risk situation we meet a fork in the road, offering the choice between learning or quitting. For this reason, you need to develop what's called a "growth mindset," which is thinking that we can learn through trial and error, and practice.

Most people who are on the journey of weight loss tell the story of having lost and regained weight many times.

One of the first questions to ask is what were the causes of the weight regain? If you can pinpoint the causes of past failures, then you can turn them to your advantage.

For example, a friend of mine who has lost 50 pounds with a combination of better eating and regular exercise; nothing unusual or extreme in her approach and it was going great…. until she fell back into her usual pattern of caring for everyone else and not making time for herself.

Thus, she reverted to her old habits of not planning or organizing her eating and not exercising, and inevitably regained the weight. In embarking on another attempt to fix her weight problem, she needed to be very clear from the start about what it will take to avoid a repetition of what happened. She will need to truly address her lifestyle issue of not making herself a priority in her own life.

In the world of business, leaders are advised to get their teams to do a "pre-mortem" before launching into a new program. The idea is to imagine that the program has failed and to think of all the reasons why it did. This is to provide insight into all the pitfalls that should be avoided. The reason this exercise is a good idea is because of the natural tendency for people to be overly optimistic when in a highly motivated state, and to ignore potential risks.

We really want to achieve the outcome, so we convince ourselves that we are bound to succeed. That's a dangerous attitude, and one which makes us more "fragile."

Proven Obesity Code

Better to start by facing the risks that lie ahead
and using our past experiences to teach us. That
is the key to relapse prevention!

Dr. Jason Fred

CHAPTER SIX

THE ROLE OF A HEALTHY MIND IN WEIGHT LOSS

A person who wants to take care of his health, will need a strong and coherent mentality. Achieving a state of well-being and mental balance helps us to produce the energy necessary to be firmer in our mental health purposes.

Having a toned body and good morale helps keep your balance, the two being closely intertwined. Physical activity strengthens the muscles as well as the mind and builds self-esteem. And a good psychic balance, a fulfilling social life stimulate the desire to work on the body and its endurance.

We often tend to attribute the right physical balance to our body, to food, to the activities we engage in... It's true, but not only! The psyche also plays an essential role. Indeed, our bodily experience and our mental health are very dependent on each other. Paying attention to your body, having an active lifestyle, playing sports, and enjoying it, it's just as good for our health as it is for our morale. It gives us a feeling of well-being, and encourages us to both optimism and action and develops our cognitive functions. Thanks to this balance, both physical and mental, we can adapt to aging, continue to feel good and, of course, avoid falls.

A good mental hygiene passes above all by a good hygiene of life. Valid in all circumstances, the rules to follow to observe a healthy lifestyle are more than ever in order. Starting with a varied and balanced diet, which leaves room for sharing and pleasure. Just as fundamental for your psychic well-being, the quality of your sleep must be the object of all the attentions.

To find serene and restful nights, get enough sleep at a fixed time, avoiding the late use of screens which disrupts our biological clock. During the day, maintain a regular rhythm and schedule as much as possible.

Eat better, sleep well... and move more! Physical activity, whose health benefits are well established, has a real antidepressant effect. Regular practice, even moderate intensity, and adapted to your physical condition, not only builds your self-confidence but also frees you from psychological tensions (thanks to the secretion of endorphins) and reduces the risk of insomnia.

Is your gym closed for health reasons? It is always possible to exercise outdoors or work out in your living room! Many online courses offer muscle building, flexibility or balance sessions, which you can take at home, without special equipment.

Beyond sport, other "soft" disciplines promote relaxation of the muscles like that of the mind. Easy to practice at home with the help of the Internet, meditation, yoga or sophrology are recognized relaxation methods, based on breath control. By amplifying breathing and therefore oxygenation of the body and brain, they help regulate our emotions and reduce stress.

The outings being authorized, apply, as soon as possible, these techniques in the open air. Take the opportunity to expose yourself to the sun, a source of vitamin D for good morale, and to daylight, which stimulates the production of serotonin, "the hormone of good mood".

And if you have the possibility, reconnect with the surrounding nature, time for a stroll. An experience by definition multisensory - view of vegetation, birdsong, scent of flowers - regular frequentation of green spaces alleviates anxiety, depression and the feeling of loneliness. Other anti-stress remedies: creative or artistic hobbies. Painting, drawing, coloring, gluing, sewing or knitting are all ways to let go, take time for yourself and put your difficulties aside for a moment.

Another way to keep the body and mind alert, to stay independent, to fight against melancholy, is to have a rich social life through various activities: community involvement, occasional volunteering, neighborhood councils, shared gardens, orchestra or choir, associative commitments or simple service to your neighbor: solidarity in all its forms strengthens the feeling of usefulness and self-esteem. Helping those who need it, many in these times of economic and social crisis, will be beneficial for you too. Indeed, it stimulates the desire to find a body balance.

Social life allows us to maintain our ability to manage relationships with others. It is about appeasing conflict situations, measuring the risks to be taken or acquiring a certain wisdom. All these social interactions have a very positive impact on our body, on self-esteem and on our mental health.

The ordeal we face collectively can also be an opportunity for personal "refocusing". This is the time to show kindness and empathy towards yourself, to listen to yourself more, to indulge yourself in small pleasures.

And, why not, cultivate your optimism! This is the principle of positive psychology, a field of scientific research which is interested in the conditions of our happiness. Focusing on what is going well - while remaining lucid - allows us to draw the positive from us and around us. And thus, to regain our capacity to act to move forward.

CHAPTER SEVEN

CONCLUSION

Setting unattainable weight loss goals is counterproductive and can even be dangerous for your health. Better to aim for a realistic weight, that you will reach serenely and for the long term and with which you feel good, whether you are thin or round.

In addition to motivation, which has been fully dealt with in this guide, as the essential element to succeed in achieving a weight loss goal, the assistance and advice of professionals remain essential elements for success in cutting down and especially for not to gain weight.

Anyone who wants to change something in their life needs motivation. It is not only by repeating the good resolutions that you have set for yourself, such as "I want to lose weight" or "I would like to do more sport" that you will get there. You need to set a smart goal. A relevant goal is the foundation of your motivation.

To lose weight effectively and safely, it is necessary to be patient and follow a healthy and balanced diet, combined with a program of regular physical activity, the duration of which should be gradually increased. This way you can lose weight while protecting your health.

Including new eating habits and regular physical exercise in your daily routine can be the beginning of the change to a healthier and more fulfilling life.

Also, to prevent or combat obesity, it is essential to pay attention to the body mass index (BMI), in addition to changing the lifestyle. In childhood or adulthood, the main risk factors for developing the problem are lack of physical activity and an unbalanced diet.

Printed in Great Britain
by Amazon

27165452R00040